The Ultimate Healthy Instant Pot Cookbook

The Instant Pot Cookbook with Healthy, and Time-Saved Recipes to Stay Your Figure While Enjoying Best Tasty Food.

Brian Smith

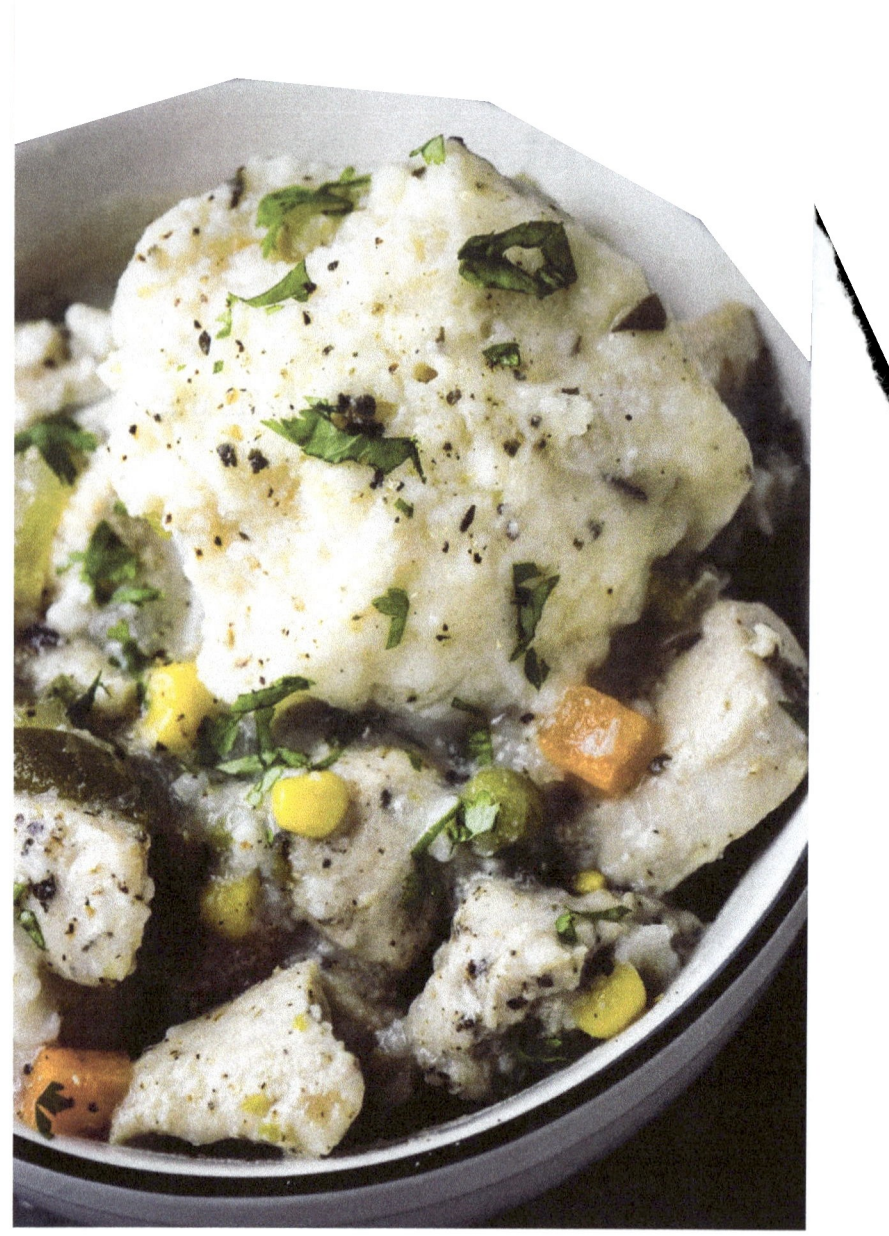

Table of Contents

scenarios in which the publisher or the original author of this work can be in any fashion deemed liable for any hardship or damages that may befall them after undertaking information described herein. Additionally, the information in the following pages is intended only for informational purposes and should thus be thought of as universal. As befitting its nature, it is presented without assurance regarding its prolonged validity or interim quality. Trademarks that are mentioned are done without written consent and can in no way be considered an endorsement from the trademark holder.

Introduction

Instant pot is a pressure cooker, also stir-fry, stew, and cook rice, cook vegetables and chicken. It's an all-in-one device, so you can season chicken and cook it in the same pan, for example. In most cases, instant pot meals can be served in less than an hour.

Cooking less time is due to the pressure cooking function that captures the steam generated by the liquid cooking environment (including liquids released from meat and vegetables), boosts the pressure and pushes the steam back.

But don't confuse with traditional pressure cookers. The instant pot, unlike the pressure cooker used by grandparents, eliminates the risk of safety with a lid that locks and remains locked until pressure is released.

Even when cooking time is over in the instant pot, you need to take an additional step-to release the pressure.

There are two ways to relieve pressure. Due to the natural pressure release, the lid valve remains in the sealing position and the pressure will naturally dissipate over time. This process takes 20 minutes to over an hour, depending on what is cooked. Low fluidity foods (such as chicken wings) take less time than high fluidity foods such as soups and marinades.

Another option is manual pressure release (also called quick release). Now you need to carefully move the valve to the ventilation position and see that the steam rises slowly and the pressure is released. This Directions is much faster, but foods with high liquid content, such as soups, take about 15 minutes to manually relieve pressure.

Which option should I use? Take into account that even if natural pressure is released, the instant pot is still under pressure. This means that the food will continue to cook while the instant pot is in sealed mode. Manual pressure relief is useful when the dishes are well cooked and need to be stopped as soon as possible.

If the goal is to prepare meals quickly, set the cooking time for dishes that are being cooked in an instant pop and release the pressure manually after the time has passed.

Instant pots (called "Instapot" by many) are one of our favorite cookware because they can handle such a wide range of foods almost easily. Instant pots range from those that work on the basics of pressure cooking to those that can be sterilized using Suicide video or some models can be controlled via Wi-Fi.

In addition, if you want to expand the range of kitchenware, the Instant Pot brand has released an air fryer that can be used to make rotisserie chicken and homemade beef jerky. There is also an independent accumulator device that can be used in instant pots to make fish, steaks and more.

The current icon instant pot works like a pressure cooker and uses heat and steam to quickly cook food. Everything from perfect carnitas to boiled eggs was cooked, but not all ingredients and DIRECTIONSs work. Here are few foods that should not be cooked in classic instant pots.

Instant pots are not pressure fryer and are not designed to handle the high temperatures required to heat cooking oils like crispy fried chicken. Of course, the instant pot is great for dishes like Carnitas, but after removing the meat from the instant pot, to get the final crispness in the meat, transfer it to a frying pan for a few minutes or to an oven top and hot Crispy in the oven.

As with slow cookers, dairy products such as cheese, milk, and sour cream will pack into instant pots using pressure cooking settings or slow cooking settings. Do not add these ingredients after the dish are cooked or create a recipe in Instapot.

There are two exceptions. One is when making yogurt. This is merely possible if you are using an instant pot recipe. The other is only when making cheesecake and following an instant pot recipe.

Although you can technically cook pasta in an instant pot, gummy may appear and cooking may be uneven. To be honest, unless you have a choice, cooking pasta in a stove pot is just as fast and easy and consistently gives you better cooked pasta.

Instead of baking the cake in an instant pot, steam it. The cake is moist-it works for things like bread pudding-but there is no good skin on the cake or on the crunchy edge everyone fights with a baked brownie. However, let's say your desire is to build a close-up or a simple dessert with your family; you can get a damp sponge in about 30 minutes, except during the DIRECTIONS time.

Canning, a technique for cooking and sealing food in a jar, is often done in a pressure cooker. Therefore, it is recommended to create a batch of jam, pickles or jelly in Instapot. Please do not.

With an instant pot, you can't monitor the temperature of what you can, like a normal pressure cooker. In canning, it is important to cook and seal the dishes correctly. Incorrect cooking and sealing can lead to the growth of bacteria that can cause food poisoning.

If you want to avoid canning in an instant pot, some newer models, such as Duo Plus, have a sterilization setting that can clean kitchen items such as baby bottles, bottles and cookware.

Instant Pot Pressure Cooker Safety Tips

Instant Pot is a very safe pressure cooker consisting of various safety mechanisms. do not worry. It will not explode immediately. Most accidents are caused by user errors and can be easily avoided. To further minimize the possibility of an accident, we have compiled a list of safety tips.

1 Don't leave it alone

It is not recommended to leave home while cooking an instant pot. If you have to leave it alone, make sure it is under pressure and no steam is coming out.

2 Do not use KFC in instant pot

Do not fry in an instant pot or other pressure cooker.

KFC uses a commercial pressure fryer specially made to fry chicken (the latest one that operates at 5 PSI). Instant pots (10.5-11.6 PSI) are specially made to make our lives easier.

3 water intake!

Instant pots require a minimum of 1 1/2 cup liquid (Instant Pot Official Number) 1 cup liquid to reach and maintain pressure.

The liquid can be a combination of gravy, vinegar, water, chicken etc.

4 half full or half empty

The max line printed on the inner pot of the instant pot is not for pressure cooking.

For pressure cooking: up to 2/3 full

Food for pressure cooking that expands during cooking (grains, beans, dried vegetables, etc.): up to 1/2

5 Not a facial steamer

Deep cleaning is not performed even if the pressure cooker steam is used once.

When opening, always tilt the lid away from you. Wear waterproof and heat-resistant silicone gloves especially when performing quick release.

6 never use power

In situations of zero, you should try to force open the lid of the instant pot pressure cooker, unless you want to prevent a light saber from hitting your face.

7 Wash Up & Checkout

If you want to be secured, wash the lid after each use and clean the anti-block shield and inner pot. Make sure that the gasket (silicon seal ring) is in good shape and that there is no food residue in the anti-block shield before use.

Usually silicone seal rings should be replaced every 18-24 months. It is always advisable to keep extra things.

Do not purchase a sealing ring from a third party because it is an integral part of the safety features of the instant ring.

Using sealing rings that have not been tested with instant pot products can create serious safety concerns."

Before use, make sure that the sealing ring is securely fixed to the sealing ring rack and the anti-block shield is properly attached to the vapor discharge pipe.

A properly fitted sealing ring can be moved clockwise or counterclockwise in the sealing ring rack with little force.

With instant pots, the whole family can cook meals in less than 30 minutes. Cooked dishes such as rice, chicken, beef stew, sauce, yakitori can be cooked for 30-60 minutes from the beginning to the end. And yes, you can bake bread in an instant pot.

Old and ketogenic diet fans love instant pots for their ability to `` roast " meat in such a short time, but vegetarians and vegans that can quickly cook dishes such as pumpkin soup, baked potatoes and marinated potato chilis, also highly appreciated oatmeal cream and macaroni and cheese.

Even dried beans, which usually require overnight cooking, can be prepared in 30 minutes to make spicy hummus.

Millet Porridge

Preparation Time: 10 minutes

Cooking Time: 9 minutes

Servings: 2

Ingredients:

1 cup of water

½ cup millet

1 ½ tablespoon honey

3 tablespoons fresh blueberries

Directions:

In the instant pot, mix together water and millet.

Make sure to lock the lid and cook at air mass for ten minutes.

After the cooking is complete, use a quick pressure release.

Remove the lid and with a fork. Fluff the porridge.

Drizzle with honey and serve with a topping of blueberries.

Nutrition:

Calories – 245

Protein – 5.7 g. Fat – 2.2 g., Carbs – 51.4 g.

Chia Spiced Rice Pudding

Preparation Time: 5 minutes

Cooking Time: 15 minutes

Servings: 2

Ingredients:

6 Medjool dates, sliced

2 tablespoons brown sugar

1 teaspoon cinnamon powder

1 cup short-grain rice

1 teaspoon ginger powder

1 cup almond milk, unsweetened

1½ cups water

1 cup coconut milk, unsweetened

¼ teaspoon nutmeg

5 cardamom pods

1 teaspoon vanilla extract

Pinch of salt

Directions:

Take your instant pot and place it on a clean kitchen platform. Turn it on after plugging it into a power socket. Open the lid from the top and put it aside; start adding the mentioned ingredients inside and gently stir them. Do not add the garnishes.

Make sure to lock the lid and lock. Make sure that you have sealed the valve to avoid leakage.

Press "Manual" mode and set a timer for 10 minutes. Wait for a few minutes for the pot to build inside pressure and start cooking.

After the timer reaches zero, press "cancel" and naturally release pressure. It takes about 8-10 minutes to naturally release pressure.

Cautiously open the lid and mix the rice. Top with the garnishes and serve warm!

Nutrition:

Calories – 242

Protein – 2.5 g.

Fat – 2 g.

Carbs – 31.5 g.

Cheesy Bacon Oats

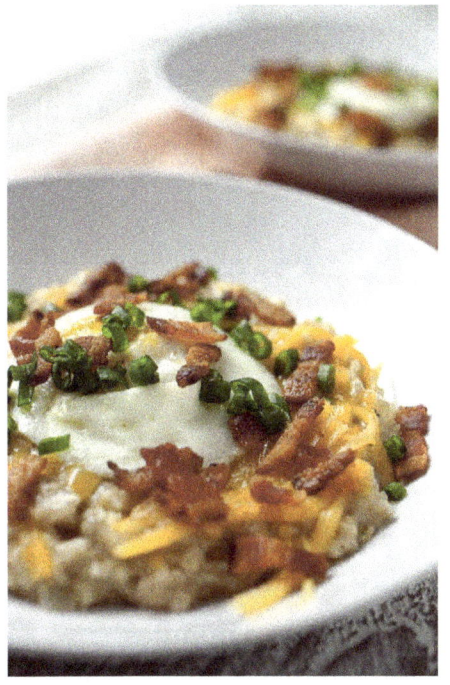

Preparation Time: 5 minutes

Cooking Time: 12 minutes

Servings: 2

Ingredients:

4 slices bacon, cooked and crumbled

1 small onion, finely chopped

¼ cup Gouda cheese, shredded

¼ cup of water

6 ounces chicken stock

½ cup steel-cut oats

1 tablespoon butter

1 tablespoon olive oil

Black pepper and salt, as needed

Directions:

Place your instant pot on a dry surface and open the lid.

Press SAUTE; add the butter and melt it.

Mix in the onion; cook for 3 minutes until soft and translucent.

Add the oats, stock, olive oil, a pinch of black pepper (ground) and salt.

Make sure to lock the lid and ensure it is sealed properly.

Press MANUAL; set timer to 9 minutes.

The instant pot will start building pressure; allow the mixture to cook for the set time.

After the timer reaches zero, wait for the float valve to drop. It will take 8-10 minutes.

Open the lid and get the oats then put it on a plate.

Divide among serving plates/bowls; serve warm.

Nutrition:

Calories – 287

Protein – 11.3 g.

Fat – 23.2 g.

Carbs – 21 g.

Crunchy Cinnamon Toast Rice Pudding

Preparation Time: 10 minutes

Cooking Time: 25 minutes

Servings: 2

Ingredients:

1 cup of water

1/8 tsp. ground cinnamon,

¼ cup of sugar

1/3 teaspoon vanilla extract

¾ cup Arborio rice

1 1/3 tablespoon maple syrup

1 ½ egg

1 1/3 cups whole milk

1 bay leaf

2 dashes ground nutmeg

Cinnamon toast crunch cereal, for topping

About 1 tablespoon eggnog, for serving, optional

Directions:

Put the rice salt, bay leaf, and water in the inner pot. Secure the lid and close the pressure valve. Fix the IP to MANUAL high pressure for 3 minutes. NPR for 10 minutes when the timer beeps, then QPR. While the rice is cooking, put the eggs, 1/3 cup milk, vanilla, cinnamon, and nutmeg in a mixing bowl. Whisk until combined well. Set aside. Open the IP lid. Remove and discard bay leaf. Add the 1 cup milk, maple syrup, and sugar; stir to combine well, scraping the bottom of the pot to dislodge stuck rice. Set a fine-mesh strainer on the IP lid.

Pour the custard mixture through a strainer. Immediately press the CANCEL key. Set the IP to SAUTE "more" mode. Mix continuously for 3-5 minutes until the mixture is bubbly and sticky. Turn the IP off. Immediately remove the inner pot from the housing and put on a heat-safe surface. This step should take 5 minutes tops. You can eat the pudding while warm. If you want it cold, let the inner pot cool. Cover and refrigerate the pudding for at least 2 to 3 hours. Serve topped with the cereal. If you want to lighten the mixture, add heavy cream, half-and-half, milk, or eggnog to your serving before topping.

Nutrition:

Calories – 420, Protein – 10 g. , Fat – 7 g., Carbs – 78 g.

Bacon Egg Mystery Muffins

Preparation Time: 5 minutes

Cooking Time: 10 minutes

Servings: 2

Ingredients:

1 cups of water

2 bacon slices, cooked and crumbled, divided

1/8 teaspoon lemon pepper seasoning

2 eggs

½ scallion, chopped and divided

2 tablespoon shredded cheddar cheese, divided

Salt to taste

Directions:

In a bowl, whip together the eggs, lemon pepper, and salt

Divide the cheese onion and bacon, between 2 silicone muffin cups.

Pour the egg mixture over.

Transfer the water into your instant pot and arrange the muffin cups on the rack.

Lock the lid, and turn the vent to: sealed"

Press "pressure cook" (manual) button, use "+" or "-"button to set the timer for 10 minutes. Use "pressure level" button to set the pressure to high.

Once done, press "Cancel" button and turns the steam release handle to "venting" position for quick release until the float valve drops down.

Open the lid. Serve and enjoy!

Nutrition:

Calories – 72

Protein – 4.3 g.

Fat – 2.6 g.

Carbs – 1.6 g.

Morning Sweet Potato Breakfast Bowls

Preparation Time: 5 minutes

Cooking Time: 20 minutes

Servings: 4

Ingredients:

4 medium sweet potatoes, cleaned

1 cup of water

A small pinch of sea salt

1/2 teaspoon of organic ground cinnamon powder

2 tablespoons of maple syrup or pure organic honey

Banana slices (Topping)

Directions:

Place a wire rack insert or a steamer basket in your Instant Pot pressure cooker.

Place the sweet potatoes on top and pour in the 1 cup of water.

Cover and seal the lid on your Instant Pot.

Choose the "Manual" button and cook for 15 minutes on High Pressure.

When the cooking is done, wait for 5 minutes before quick-releasing the pressure and removing the lid.

Carefully remove the sweet potatoes.

Scoop the sweet potato flesh away from the skin and place to a bowl.

Add the salt, cinnamon powder, and honey. Mash until reached your desired consistency.

Top with banana slices.

Serve and enjoy!

Nutrition:

Calories – 293

Protein – 9.6 g.

Fat – 0.5 g.

Carbs – 69.3 g.

Optimum Chicken and Apple Meatballs

Preparation Time: 5 minutes

Cooking Time: 20 minutes

Servings: 4

Ingredients:

1-1/2 pound of ground chicken

3 tablespoons of coconut oil

1 apple, peeled, cored and sliced to small pieces

2 tablespoons of dried oregano

2 tablespoons of dried thyme

2 tablespoons of dried parsley

1 teaspoon of garlic powder

1/2 teaspoon of sea salt

1/2 teaspoon of fresh black pepper

1/4 cup of homemade low-sodium chicken broth or water

Directions:

Press the "Sauté" function on your Instant Pot and add 1 tablespoon of coconut oil.

Add the finely chopped apples to the Instant Pot along with the dried herbs. Sauté for 6 to 8 minutes or until softened, stirring occasionally.

Remove the apples from the Instant Pot and turn off.

In a bowl, mix the chicken with the apples, garlic powder, salt, and black pepper.

Form the mixture into meatballs.

Press the "Sauté" function on your Instant Pot and add the remaining 2 tablespoons of coconut oil.

If necessary, working in batches, add the meatballs and cook until no longer pink.

Add the chicken broth.

Close and seal the lid. Choose the "Manual" button and cook for 5 minutes at High Pressure.

When the timer beeps, quick release or naturally release the pressure and remove the lid.

Serve and enjoy!

Nutrition:

Calories – 412

Protein – 26 g.

Fat – 30 g.

Carbs – 15 g.

Gratifying Kale Butternut Squash and Pancetta Breakfast Hash

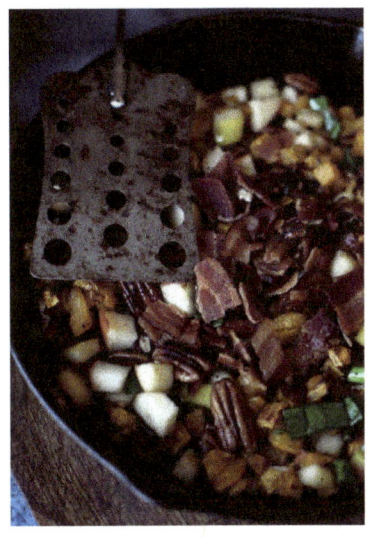

Preparation Time: 5 minutes

Cooking Time: 30 minutes

Servings: 6

Ingredients:

1 lb. of butternut squash, sliced into small cubes

1 large bunch of fresh kale, roughly chopped

2 garlic cloves, minced

1/2 medium onion, finely chopped

4 medium bacon slices, thickly sliced

1 tbsp. of olive oil or coconut oil

1/4 cup of water or low-sodium vegetable broth

2 teaspoons of apple cider vinegar

1 teaspoon of sea salt

1 teaspoon of freshly cracked black pepper

Directions:

Press the "Sauté" function on your Instant Pot and add the oil.

Once hot and ready, add the bacon and cook until brown and crispy, stirring occasionally. Remove and set aside

Add the squash cubes, garlic, and onion to your Instant Pot. Sauté until lightly tender, stirring occasionally.

Stir in the roughly chopped kale, vegetable broth, and apple cider vinegar to your Instant Pot.

Let it cook until the liquid is reduced, the squash is tender, and the kale has wilted, typically around 5 minutes.

Stir in the bacon, sea salt, and freshly cracked black pepper.

Serve and enjoy!

Nutrition:

Calories – 169

Protein – 6.9 g.

Fat – 7.7 g.

Carbs – 14.6 g.

Palatable Maple Bacon Banana Breakfast Muffins

Preparation Time: 5 minutes
Cooking Time: 30 minutes
Servings: 6
Ingredients:

3 large ripe bananas, mashed

2-1/2 cups of coconut flour

1 teaspoon of baking soda

1/4 cup of maple syrup

6 medium bacon slices, cooked and finely chopped

1/2 cup of unsweetened coconut yogurt

1/2 cup of unsweetened coconut milk

A small pinch of sea salt

Directions:

Grease individual muffin cups or ramekins with nonstick cooking spray.

In a large bowl,put the coconut flour, mashed bananas, baking soda, maple syrup, bacon slices, coconut yogurt, coconut milk, and sea salt.

Gently stir until fully combined.

Split and pour the batter into the muffin cups or ramekins.

Add 1 cup of water and a trivet to your Instant Pot.

Place the muffin cups or ramekins on top of the trivet.
Cover and seal the lid. Cook at High Pressure for 25
minutes.

Once done, naturally release pressure for 10 minutes
before quick releasing the remaining pressure.

Remove the muffins and allow to cool.

Serve and enjoy!

Nutrition:

Calories – 396

Protein – 18 g.

Fat – 16.9 g.

Carbs – 50.3 g.

Highly Regarded Cauliflower and Sweet Potato Breakfast Hash

Preparation Time: 5 minutes

Cooking Time: 20 minutes

Servings: 6

Ingredients:

6 large sweet potatoes

1 large cauliflower head, cut into florets

1 large onion, finely chopped

2 tbsp. of coconut oil or olive oil

6 medium bacon slices, finely diced

3 garlic cloves, minced

1/2 cup of homemade low-sodium vegetable stock

2 teaspoons of freshly squeezed lemon juice

3 tablespoons of fresh rosemary

3 tablespoons of fresh basil

1 teaspoon of sea salt

1 teaspoon of freshly cracked black pepper

Directions:

Press the "Sauté" function on your Instant Pot and add the oil.

Once the oil is hot and ready, add the garlic and onions.

Sauté until softened, stirring occasionally.

Add the sweet potatoes and cauliflower to the Instant Pot.

Add the bacon to the Instant Pot along with the salt, black pepper, rosemary, and basil. Sauté for a few minutes, stirring occasionally.

Add the vegetable stock and lemon juice to the Instant Pot.

Cover and cook on High Pressure for 10 minutes.

When the cooking is done, quick release or naturally release the pressure. Remove the lid.

Drain the liquid and transfer the vegetables to a serving bowl.

Serve and enjoy!

Nutrition:

Calories – 353

Protein – 12.1 g.

Fat – 12.9 g.

Carbs – 49.5 g.

Instant Pot Asparagus and Goat Cheese Frittatas

Preparation Time: 10 minutes

Cooking Time: 50 minutes

Servings: 4

Ingredients:

8 ounces of asparagus, trimmed and sliced

1 Red bell pepper, medium, stemmed and chopped

2 shallots, minced

½ cup of goat cheese, crumbled

1 tablespoon fresh tarragon, grated

1 teaspoon lemon zest, grated

8 eggs, large

1 tablespoon olive oil

½ teaspoon of salt

Directions:

Add some oil in the Instant Pot in SAUTE mode and wait for the unit display shows HOT.

When the oil becomes hot, add the bell pepper, Asparagus, shallots and cook it until it becomes soft, it should take about 5 minutes.

Transfer the vegetables to another bowl when cooked.

Add the goat cheese, lemon zest, and tarragon in the same bowl and mix it to make the ramekins.

Place the trivet in the Instant Pot, which comes with the Instant Pot and pour 1 cup of water in the Instant Pot. Spray the ramekins with the vegetable oil.

In another bowl, beat the eggs, ¼ cup water, and salt together until it combined well.

Divide the vegetable mixture equally between the ramekins and then pour the egg mixture on top of them. Keep the mixture filled ramekins on the trivet and close the instant pot.

Choose Pressure Cook mode and cook for 10 minutes in HIGH PRESSURE.

When done, turn on the QUICK RELEASE valve.

After releasing the pressure, remove the lid and let the steam escape from the pot entirely.

Transfer the dish into the wire rack and cut it using the paring knife when it has cooled down.

Cut around the inside's edges of the ramekins to get the frittatas loosened up from the sides.

Serve it as needed.

Nutrition:

Calories – 288

Protein – 15 g.

Fat – 21.5 g.

Carbs – 9 g.

Instant Pot Black Rice Pudding

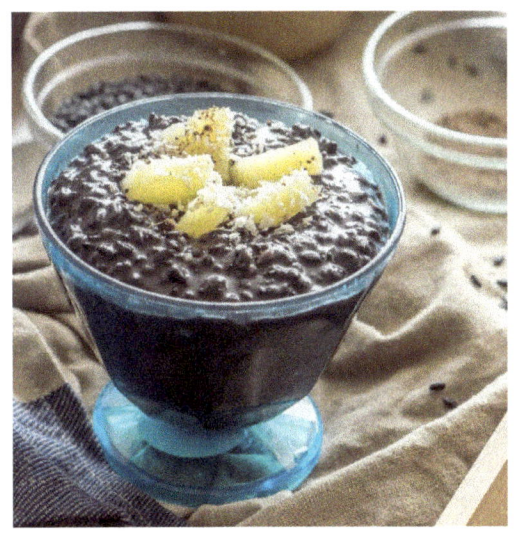

Preparation Time: 5 minutes

Cooking Time: 60 minutes

Servings: 4

Ingredients:

1 cup of Indonesian black rice

14 ounces can of coconut milk, full fat

2 tablespoons coconut sugar

½ cup banana

½ cup coconut chips

½ cup hemp hearts

½ teaspoon salt

1½ cup of water

Directions:

Mix the coconut milk, coconut sugar, black rice, and 1 cup of water in the Instant Pot and close the lid.

Lock the pressure vent too.

At MANUAL settings, Put the instant potat HIGH PRESSURE for 22 minutes.

Once the cooking is done, naturally release the pressure for 10 minutes.

Remove the lid and stir the rice pudding well.

Garnish with coconut chips, bananas, and hemp hearts while serving.

Serve hot.

Nutrition:

Calories – 251

Protein – 6 g.

Fat – 10.8 g.

Carbs – 43 g.

Broccoli Frittata with Ham and Peppers

Preparation Time: 10 minutes

Cooking Time: 30 minutes

Servings: 4

Ingredients:

8 ounces of ham, cubed

1 cup sweet pepper, sliced

2 cups broccoli, frozen

4 eggs, medium

1 cup of Half and Half

1 cup cheddar cheese, shredded

1 teaspoon salt

2 teaspoons pepper, ground

Directions:

Grease an Instant Pot insert pan thoroughly.

Put the sliced sweet peppers at the bottom of the pan, followed by the cubed ham on top.

Cover the dish with broccoli.

Using a mixing bowl, whisk the eggs, salt, pepper, and Half and Half together.

Add some shredded cheese and stir well.

Pour this mixture over the vegetables and ham and cover with foil.

Pour two cups of water in the Instant Pot and place a trivet.

Place the covered broccoli frittata on the trivet.

Choose "pressure cook manual" mode and set the timer for 20 minutes at HIGH PRESSURE.

After 20 minutes, let the pressure release naturally.

Using a knife, loosen the dish and layout the frittata on a plate and serve it with some cheese over the dish.

Nutrition:

Calories – 279

Protein – 26 g.

Fat – 12.4 g.

Carbs – 16 g.

Instant Pot Chocolate Quinoa Breakfast Bowl

Preparation Time: 10 minutes

Cooking Time: 10 minutes

Servings: 6

Ingredients:

1 butter slab, silver

1 cup quinoa

1 can coconut milk

1 tablespoon cocoa powder

½ teaspoon hazelnut extract

2 tablespoon maple syrup

⅓ cup milk

Fruit toppings as desired

Directions:

In the SAUTE MODE, melt some butter in the Instant Pot. When the butter becomes hot, add the quinoa and stir until it coats the butter well and toasted.

Once done, add the other ingredients in the pot and stir it well as it cooks.

Once the cocoa powder mixes thoroughly with the mixture, close the lid.

Change the cooking setting to MANUAL PRESSURE COOK by increasing the temperature at HIGH and timer for 2 minutes, set the vent to 'SEALING,' and let it cook. After the timer elapsed, release the pressure manually for about 5 minutes.

Serve it warm with desired toppings.

Nutrition:

Calories – 240

Protein – 5 g.

Fat – 13.9 g.

Carbs – 25 g.

Corn Meal Porridge in Instant Pot

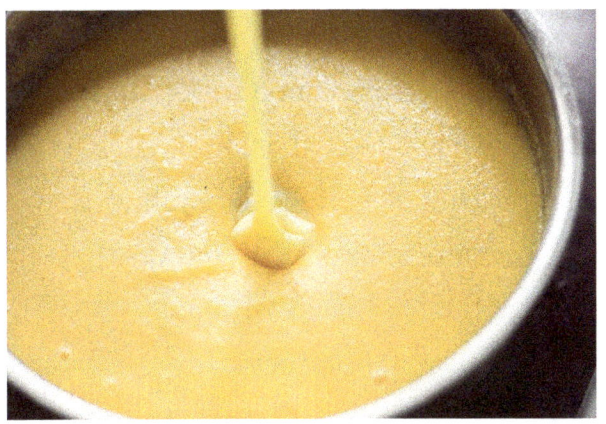

Preparation Time: 5 minutes

Cooking Time: 20 minutes

Servings: 4

Ingredients:

1 cup of yellow cornmeal, fine

2 sticks of cinnamon

2 pimento berries

½ teaspoon nutmeg, ground

1 teaspoon vanilla extract

½ cup condensed milk, sweetened

4 cups of water

1 cup milk

Directions:

Pour the milk and 3 cups of water in the Instant Pot.

In a medium bowl, mix well the cornmeal with 1 cup water.

Transfer this mixture into the Instant Pot while you continue to stir.

Now add the berries, nutmeg, cinnamon sticks, vanilla extract in the Instant Pot, and close the lid.

Cook the mixture on PORRIDGE mode for 6 minutes.

When done, let the pressure release for 10 minutes naturally.

Whisk it well to avoid any lumps and serve it warm with some condensed milk.

Nutrition:

Calories – 209

Protein – 6 g.

Fat – 3.8 g.

Carbs – 37 g.

Eggs and Cocotte in the Instant Pot

Preparation Time: 15 minutes

Cooking Time: 2 minutes

Servings: 3

Ingredients:

½ cup butter

3 tablespoons of cream

3 eggs, medium

1 tablespoon chives

1 teaspoon salt

1 teaspoon pepper, ground

1 cup of water

Directions:

Rub some butter in the inside wall of the ramekins.

Pour 1 tablespoon of butter in each ramekin.

Crack the egg and pour one egg per ramekins without breaking the yolks.

Sprinkle some chives over the eggs.

Put the trivet rack in the Instant Pot and pour a cup of water in the pot.

The amount of water should be below the rack.

Make sure to lock the lid and cook at LOW-PRESSURE COOK MODE for 2 minutes.

Set the temperature of the pot to low heat.

After cooking, release the pressure manually.

Use a kitchen towel or hot pad to remove the ramekins.

Season with salt and ground pepper, serve hot.

Nutrition:

Calories – 370

Protein – 7 g.

Fat – 37.8 g.

Carbs – 2 g.

Instant Pot Ground Corn Breakfast Bowls

Preparation Time: 10 minutes
Cooking Time: 25 minutes
Servings: 4
Ingredients:

1 cup cornmeal, stone-ground

1 cup of milk, reduce fat

1 tablespoon canola oil

½ teaspoon Worcestershire sauce

⅛ teaspoon red pepper, ground

3¾ cups water

1 garlic clove

½ teaspoon salt

Directions:

Mix the cornmeal, 2 cups of water, oil, milk, and garlic in a medium bowl.

Pour the remaining water in the Instant Pot.

Put your trivet rack in the Instant Pot.

Put the cornmeal mix in 4-cup glassware on top of the rack, inside the Instant Pot.

Make sure to lock the lid and on MANUAL PRESSURE COOK setting, and set the timer for 25 minutes in HIGH PRESSURE.

Naturally release the pressure once cooked.

Stir in some salt, pepper, and Worcestershire sauce and add ¾ cup cheese melts in the mix.

Spoon out the grits from the cooker and garnish with scallions and cheese.

Serve while it is warm.

Nutrition:

Calories – 215

Protein – 5 g.

Fat – 6.2 g.

Carbs – 35 g.

Instant Pot Apple Cinnamon French Toast Casserole

Preparation Time: 10 minutes

Cooking Time: 25 minutes

Servings: 5

Ingredients:

4 cups of whole-grain bread, bite-sized cubed

1 cup apple, chopped, skinless

¼ cup raisins

¼ cup pecans, chopped

3 eggs, medium

¼ cup applesauce

2 teaspoon apple pie spice

½ cup milk

½ teaspoon salt

Non-stick cooking spray

Directions:

Slightly grease the springform or baking pan using a nonstick cooking spray.

Combine the bread cubes, raisins, and apples in a large bowl.

In a bowl, whip the eggs with milk, apple pie spice, apple sauce, and salt and pour this mix over the bread cubes to coat thoroughly.

Add the ingredients in the baking pan.

Add a cup of water and place the trivet in the instant pot and place the baking pan on the trivet.

Secure the lid of the Instant Pot and lock the pressure valve too.

Select HIGH PRESSURE COOK in the MANUAL mode.

Set the cooking time for about 25 minutes.

After cooking, quick release the pressure and carefully remove the pan from the pot.

Serve it warm with maple syrup or desired toppings.

Nutrition:

Calories – 201

Protein – 10 g.

Fat – 11.2 g.

Carbs – 16 g.

Instant Pot Banana Bread

Preparation Time: 15 minutes

Cooking Time: 50 minutes

Servings: 12

Ingredients:

2¼ cups of overripe banana, mashed

2 cups all-purpose flour

½ teaspoon nutmeg

½ cup butter

¼ cup brown sugar

2 eggs, large, beaten

1 teaspoon vanilla extract

1 teaspoon cinnamon

¼ teaspoon salt

1 teaspoon baking soda

¼ cup white sugar

Directions:

Whisk the baking soda, flour, salt and nutmeg in a large bowl

Using another bowl, combine the butter with brown and white sugar and create a creamy texture.

Add the eggs, cinnamon, and mashed bananas in the same bowl and blend it well.

Now transfer the banana-egg mixture into the flour bowl and combine well.

Drizzle the pan with cooking spray and put the batter.

Place the stand in the Instant Pot and pour one cup water in the Instant Pot.

Cover the pan with foil and put it in the pot over the trivet.

Make sure to lock the lid and set the timer at 50 minutes in MANUAL PRESSURE COOK settings.

After cooking, use the quick-release valve to de-pressure the cooker.

Remove the pan carefully and place it on a plate or dry surface.

Cut and serve warm.

Nutrition:

Calories – 259

Protein – 5 g.

Fat – 10.7 g.

Carbs – 38 g.

Instant Pot Breakfast Burritos

Preparation Time: 15 minutes

Cooking Time: 30 minutes

Servings: 6

Ingredients:

8 eggs, large

½ cup of Half & half

½ teaspoon of coarse salt

½ teaspoon garlic powder

2 tablespoon chives, chopped

¼ cup of onions, diced

¾ cup cheese, shredded

1 cup ham, cooked and cubed

½ cup red bell pepper, diced

1 cup potato, diced

1 cup flour tortillas

¼ teaspoon pepper

Cooking spray

Directions:

Pour 1½ cups of water in the Instant Pot and set the pot to PRESSURE COOK mode.

Spray some cooking in the PIP pan that you will use for cooking.

Whisk the eggs and the Half and Half together in a medium bowl.

Add the remaining ingredients in the same bowl and transfer it into the PIP pan and cover it well using aluminum foil.

Place the pot in the Instant Pot and set the timer for 30 minutes.

Press START to begin cooking.

When cooked, let the pressure release naturally.

Remove the PIP pan from the pot carefully and discard the foil.

Gently stir and break the mixture to create the breakfast burritos.

Wrap some of the egg mixtures in flour tortillas and wrap it in a foil to refrigerate until you're ready to serve.

Nutrition:

Calories – 307

Protein – 20 g.

Fat – 19.1 g.

Carbs – 13 g.

Instant Pot Breakfast Potatoes

Preparation Time: 20 minutes

Cooking Time: 15 minutes

Servings: 5

Ingredients:

5 red potatoes, diced into ½-inch cubes

1 tablespoon nutritional yeast

2 tablespoons garlic powder

1 teaspoon of onion powder

¼ teaspoon paprika

1 onion, small

1 green bell pepper, small

3 tablespoons coconut oil

¾ cup of water

1 teaspoon salt

1 teaspoon pepper

Directions:

Combine the seasoning in one bowl and set it aside.

Put the potatoes and pour oil into the Instant Pot and select the SAUTÉ feature.

Put the timer for 5 minutes and press START to begin the sauté cooking.

Stir continuously by flipping the potatoes for 5 minutes.

Once the potatoes start to change the texture, add the seasoning and continue stirring.

When the potatoes cooked well, press CANCEL/STOP to cease cooking.

Pour water into the Instant Pot.

Make sure to lock the lid and change the temperature to the LOW setting for 1 minute.

When done, gently mix the potatoes and do not mash it.

Refrigerate for 2 hours or overnight.

Before serving, remove it from the refrigerator.

Warm the potato mix by pouring oil in the Instant Pot in SAUTE mode. Set the temperature low for 10 minutes and press START.

When the oil becomes warm, add potatoes and other veggies and continue stirring.

Once the potatoes turs crispy and the vegetables get tender, serve immediately.

Nutrition:

Calories – 363

Protein – 9 g. Fat – 8.8 g. Carbs – 66 g.

Instant Pot Chocolate Chip Banana Bread Bites

Preparation Time: 10 minutes

Cooking Time: 35 minutes

Servings: 14

Ingredients:

3 bananas, extra ripe, mashed

1 egg, beaten

1 teaspoon vanilla extract

½ cup dark chocolate chips

1½ cups of flour

1 teaspoon baking soda

½ teaspoon salt

½ cup white sugar

⅓ cup butter, melted

1 cup of water

Directions:

Mix the melted butter, vanilla, egg, and sugar in a medium bowl.

Add the mashed bananas and keep stirring.

Now put baking soda and chocolate chips in the mixture.

Continue stirring when you add new items.

Transfer this mixture in the silicone molds until ¾ full and cover it with aluminum foil.

Pour a cup of water in the Instant Pot.

Put a trivet in the Instant Pot.

Place the mold on the trivet and stack the remaining on top of each other.

Close the lid properly and cook on PRESSURE COOK mode at high temperature for 25 minutes.

Press START to begin the cooking.

Once cooked, allow it to release the pressure for 10 minutes naturally.

Take off the foils and remove the molds.

Serve warm.

Nutrition:

Calories – 242,Protein – 4 g., Fat – 7.9 g.

Carbs – 42 g.

Instant Pot Congee

Preparation Time: 10 minutes

Cooking Time: 35 minutes

Servings: 6

Ingredients:

1 cup of jasmine rice

1 tablespoon canola oil

6 pieces of chicken drumsticks

½ cup fried shallots

1 green onion, medium, chopped

½ cup shredded chicken

8 cups of water

3 garlic pods, minced

1-inch ginger, peeled and sliced

½ tablespoon salt

1 teaspoon cilantro leaves

Directions:

To begin with, clean the rice separately.

In the meantime, in a large bowl, boil 5 cups of water with chicken drumsticks.

Let it boil until the foam rises to the top.

Take out the chicken drumsticks from the pot and also remove residue.

Put the instant potat SAUTÉ mode and add 1 tablespoon of oil.

Wait for the HOT display appear in the unit.

Put the garlic and sauté until it starts to release the fragrance.

Put the cooked chicken in the pot with 8 cups of water, ginger, and rice.

Close the lid.

Choose Pressure Cook MANUAL mode on HIGH PRESSURE.

Set the timer for 20 minutes.

Press START to begin the cooking.

After cooking, let the pressure release naturally before you open the lid.

To control the consistency, change the pot settings to SAUTÉ and continue stirring the mixture.

Season with some salt, as needed.

Shred the chicken.

Garnish with shredded chicken, green onions, and other toppings over the rice.

Serve warm.

Nutrition:

Calories – 255

Protein – 31 g. Fat – 11.4 g., Carbs – 12 g.

Instant Pot Easy Poached Egg

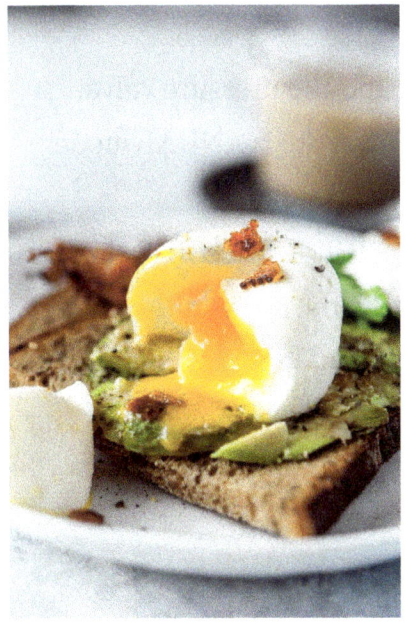

Preparation Time: 3 minutes

Cooking Time: 6 minutes

Servings: 6

Ingredients:

6 eggs, medium

½ teaspoon salt

½ teaspoon pepper

Non-stick cooking oil spray

Directions:

Pour a cup of water to the Instant Pot and place the trivet in it.

Spray the silicone tray with some nonstick cooking oil

Crack the eggs into the tray and place them on top of the trivet.

Lock the lid of the Instant Pot and the pressure valve.

Select HIGH PRESSURE COOK in the MANUAL mode.

Select the cooking time for 8 minutes.

After finish cooking, use the QUICK RELEASE option, to de-pressure the cooker and check the eggs.

Gently scoop out the eggs and sprinkle with salt and pepper.

Serve warm.

Nutrition:

Calories – 131

Protein – 9 g.

Fat – 9.7 g.

Carbs – 1 g.

Instant Pot Khaman Dhokla Recipe

Preparation Time: 10 minutes

Cooking Time: 20 minutes

Servings: 2

Ingredients:

2 cups of chickpea flour

1 teaspoon green chilies, chopped

1 teaspoon baking soda

1 teaspoon mustard seeds

1 teaspoon urad dal

2 chilies, halved

8 curry leaves

1 tablespoon coconut, grated

½ cup cilantro, chopped

2 teaspoons oil

1 tablespoon lemon juice, freshly squeezed

½ teaspoon ginger, grated

1 teaspoon sugar

1 teaspoon salt

1 teaspoon turmeric

2 cups of water

Directions:

Add all the batter ingredients in a bowl except baking soda.

Whisk to make a smooth batter, and maintain the consistency like a pancake.

Now add the baking soda and keep stirring while it develops bubbles.

Grease the mold and place the batter in the mold.

Pour the water in the Instant Pot.

Place the stand in the Instant Pot and select the function to SAUTE mode.

Continue heating until the water starts to release steam.

Transfer the mold on the trivet and close the lid.

Select HIGH PRESSURE COOK in the MANUAL mode and set the cooking time for 15 minutes.

After cooking, let the pressure release naturally.

Do a toothpick test on the dish and see if it comes clean.

Set aside for a bit and serve it warm with desired sides.

Nutrition:

Calories – 419,Protein – 21 g. Fat – 11.2 g.,
Carbs – 58 g.

Sausage Egg Breakfast

Preparation Time: 5-10 min.

Cooking Time: 12 min.

Servings: 2

Ingredients:

2 sausages, chopped

1 yellow onion, chopped

4 eggs

1 bacon slice, chopped

Directions:

In a mixing bowl, beat the eggs. Add other ingredients and stir to combine.

Grease a baking pan with some cooking spray. Add mixture over the pan.

Place Instant Vortex over the kitchen platform.

Arrange to drip pan in the lower position. Press "Air Fry," set the timer to 12 minutes, and set the temperature to 320°F. Instant Vortex will start pre-heating.

When Instant Vortex is pre-heated, it will display "Add Food" on its screen. Open the door and take out the middle roasting tray.

Place the pan over the tray and push it back; close door and cooking will start. Midway, it will display "Turn Food" on its screen; ignore it, and it will continue to cook after 10 seconds.

Open the door after the cooking cycle is over; slice and serve warm.

Nutrition:

Calories: 319

Fat: 22g

Saturated Fat: 7.5g

Trans Fat: 0.5g

Carbohydrates: 7g

Fiber: 1.5g

Sodium: 611mg

Protein: 23g

Stuffed Breakfast Peppers

Preparation Time: 5-10 min.

Cooking Time: 13 min.

Servings: 2

Ingredients:

1 bell pepper seeds removed, halved

4 eggs

Salt and black pepper to taste

¼ teaspoon red chili flakes

Directions:

Take bell peppers halves and crack two eggs into each. Season with spices on top.

Place Instant Vortex over the kitchen platform.

Arrange to drip pan in the lower position. Press "Air Fry," set the timer to 12 minutes, and set the temperature to 390°F. Instant Vortex will start pre-heating.

When Instant Vortex is pre-heated, it will display "Add Food" on its screen. Open the door and take out the middle roasting tray.

Place peppers with egg side on top over the tray and push it back; close door and cooking will start.

Midway, it will display "Turn Food" on its screen; ignore it, and it will continue to cook after 10 seconds.

Open the door after the cooking cycle is over; serve warm.

Nutrition:

Calories: 173, Fat: 12g , Saturated Fat: 2.5g , Trans Fat: 0g Carbohydrates: 6g, Fiber: 0.5g, Sodium: 350mg , Protein: 11g

Healthy Ham Egg Omelet

Preparation Time: 5-10 min.

Cooking Time: 10 min.

Servings: 4

Ingredients:

1 medium red bell pepper, deseeded and chopped

1 medium green bell pepper, deseeded and chopped

¾ cup cooked ham, chopped

8 eggs

1 cup whole milk

Ground black pepper and salt to taste

½ tablespoon chopped chives

½ cup grated cheddar cheese

½ cup chopped scallions

Directions:

In a mixing bowl, beat the eggs. Add other ingredients. Combine the ingredients to mix well with each other. Grease a baking pan with some cooking spray. Place egg mixture over the pan.

Place Instant Vortex over the kitchen platform. Arrange to drip pan in the lower position. Press "Air Fry," set the timer to 10 minutes, and set the temperature to 350°F. Instant Vortex will start pre-heating.

When Instant Vortex is pre-heated, it will display "Add Food" on its screen. Open the door and take out the middle roasting tray.

Place the pan over the tray and push it back; close door and cooking will start. Midway, it will display "Turn Food" on its screen; ignore it, and it will continue to cook after 10 seconds.

Open the door after the cooking cycle is over; slice and serve warm.

Nutrition:

Calories: 321

Fat: 19g

Saturated Fat: 6.5g

Trans Fat: 0g

Carbohydrates: 14

Fiber: 1.5g

Sodium: 258mg

Protein: 21g

Mushroom Frittata

Preparation Time: 5-10 min.

Cooking Time: 15 min.

Servings: 3-4

Ingredients:

¼ cup sliced tomato

¼ cup sliced mushrooms

1 cup egg white

2 tablespoon whole milk

2 tablespoon chopped chives

Ground black pepper and salt to taste

Directions:

In a mixing bowl, add mushrooms and other ingredients. Combine the ingredients to mix well with each other.

Grease a baking pan or casserole dish with some cooking spray. Place mushroom mixture over the pan. Place Instant Vortex over the kitchen platform. Arrange to drip pan in the lower position. Press "Bake," set timer to 15 minutes, and set the temperature to 320°F. Instant Vortex will start pre-heating.

When Instant Vortex is pre-heated, it will display "Add Food" on its screen. Open the door and take out the middle roasting tray.

Place the pan over the tray and push it back; close door and cooking will start. Midway, it will display "Turn Food" on its screen; ignore it, and it will continue to cook after 10 seconds. Bake until frittata is well set. Open the door after the cooking cycle is over; serve warm.

Nutrition:

Calories: 118

Fat: 6g

Saturated Fat: 1.5g

Trans Fat: 0g

Carbohydrates: 1.5g

Fiber: 0.5g

Sodium: 92mg , Protein: 8g

Spinach Bacon Quiche

Preparation Time: 5-10 min.

Cooking Time: 10 min.

Servings: 4

Ingredients:

¼ cup mozzarella cheese, shredded

½ cup Parmesan cheese, shredded

2 cooked bacon slices, chopped

½ cup spinach, chopped

2 tablespoons milk

Salt and ground black pepper, to taste

2 dashes Tabasco sauce

Directions:

In a mixing bowl, add all ingredients. Combine the ingredients to mix well with each other.

Grease a baking pan with some cooking spray. Place mixture over the pan.

Place Instant Vortex over the kitchen platform. Arrange to drip pan in the lower position. Press "Air Fry," set the timer to 10 minutes, and set the temperature to 320°F. Instant Vortex will start pre-heating.

When Instant Vortex is pre-heated, it will display "Add Food" on its screen. Open the door and take out the middle roasting tray.

Place the pan over the tray and push it back; close door and cooking will start. Midway, it will display "Turn Food" on its screen; ignore it, and it will continue to cook after 10 seconds.

Open the door after the cooking cycle is over; slice into wedges and serve warm.

Nutrition:

Calories: 143

Fat: 10g

Saturated Fat: 4.5g

Trans Fat: 0.5g

Carbohydrates: 3g

Fiber: 0.5g

Sodium: 507mg

Protein: 11g

Roasted Potato Cubes

Preparation Time: 5-10 min.

Cooking Time: min.

Servings: 2

Ingredients:

½ teaspoon smoked paprika

½ teaspoon garlic powder

5 medium potatoes, peeled and cut to 1-inch cubes

1 tablespoon olive oil

Ground black pepper and salt to taste

1 tablespoon chopped scallions

Directions:

In a mixing bowl, add potato cubes and other ingredients except for scallions. Combine the ingredients to mix well with each other.

Place Instant Vortex over the kitchen platform. Arrange to drip pan in the lower position. Press "Air Fry," set the timer to 15 minutes, and set the temperature to 400°F. Instant Vortex will start pre-heating.

In the rotisserie basket, add potato mixture.

When Instant Vortex is pre-heated, it will display "Add Food" on its screen. Open the door and lock the basket. Press the red lever and arrange the basket on the left side; now, just simply rest the basket rod over the right side.

Close door and press "Rotate"; cooking will start. Cook until potatoes are brown and crisp.

Open the door after the cooking cycle is over; serve warm with scallions on top.

Nutrition:

Calories: 208

Fat: 13g

Saturated Fat: 2g

Trans Fat: 0g

Carbohydrates: 22g

Fiber: 2g

Sodium: 94mg

Protein: 3g

Cheese Eggs Breakfast

Preparation Time: 5-10 min.

Cooking Time: 15 min.

Servings: 4

Ingredients:

1 cup grated Parmesan cheese

1 cup grated Monterey Jack cheese

½ cup all-purpose flour

1 tablespoon butter, melted

12 eggs, beaten

1 teaspoon salt

Directions:

In a mixing bowl, beat the eggs and butter. Add other ingredients. Combine the ingredients to mix well with each other.

Grease a baking pan with some cooking spray. Place egg mixture over the pan.

Place Instant Vortex over the kitchen platform. Arrange to drip pan in the lower position. Press "Bake," set timer to 15 minutes, and set the temperature to 350°F. Instant Vortex will start pre-heating.

When Instant Vortex is pre-heated, it will display "Add Food" on its screen. Open the door and take out the middle roasting tray.

Place the pan over the tray and push it back; close door and cooking will start. Midway, it will display "Turn Food" on its screen; ignore it, and it will continue to cook after 10 seconds.

Open the door after the cooking cycle is over; serve warm.

Nutrition:

Calories: 524

Fat: 31g

Saturated Fat: 9.5g

Trans Fat: 0g

Carbohydrates: 17g

Fiber: 0.5g

Sodium: 1249mg

Protein: 39g

Breakfast Salmon Patties

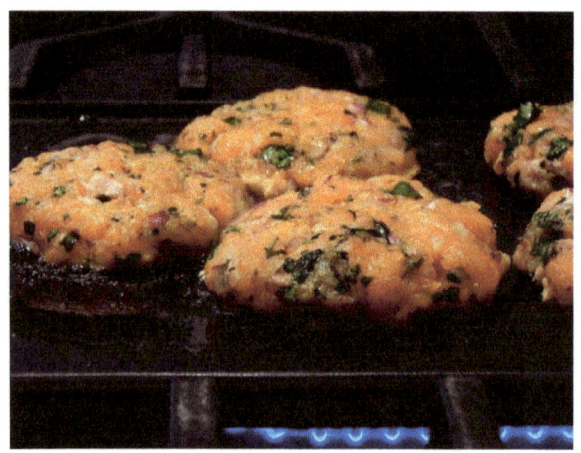

Preparation Time: 10 minutes

Cooking Time: 8 minutes

Servings: 6

Ingredients:

14 oz can salmon, drained and minced

1 tsp paprika

2 tbsp green onion, minced

2 tbsp fresh coriander, chopped

1 egg, lightly beaten

Pepper

Salt

Directions:

Preheat the instant vortex air fryer to 360 F.

Add all ingredients into the mixing bowl and mix until well combined.

Spray air fryer oven pan with cooking spray.

Make six even shape patties from salmon mixture and place on pan and air fry for 6-8 minutes. Turn halfway through.

Serve and enjoy.

Nutrition:
Calories 122
Fat 5.6 g
Carbohydrates 0.4 g
Sugar 0.2 g
Protein 16.5 g
Cholesterol 56 mg

Zucchini Fries

Preparation Time: 10 minutes

Cooking Time: 10 minutes

Servings: 4

Ingredients:

2 medium zucchinis, cut into fry's shape

½ tsp garlic powder

1 tsp Italian seasoning

½ cup parmesan cheese, grated

½ cup breadcrumbs

1 egg, lightly beaten

Pepper

Salt

Directions:

In a shallow bowl, mix together breadcrumbs, parmesan cheese, Italian seasoning, garlic powder, pepper, and salt.

Coat zucchini pieces with egg then coat with breadcrumb mixture.

Spray air fryer oven tray with cooking spray.

Arrange coated zucchini fries on a tray and air fry at 400 F for 10 minutes.

Serve and enjoy.

Nutrition:
Calories 240
Fat 11.3 g
Carbohydrates 13.5 g
Sugar 2.8 g
Protein 16.5 g
Cholesterol 72 mg

Breakfast Stuffed Peppers

Preparation Time: 10 minutes

Cooking Time: 13 minutes

Servings: 2

Ingredients:

4 eggs

1 bell pepper, halved and seed removed

¼ tsp red chili flakes

Pepper

Salt

Directions:

Crack 2 eggs into each bell pepper half and season with pepper and salt.

Sprinkle red chili flakes on top.

Arrange peppers on air fryer oven tray and cook at 390 F for 13 minutes.

Serve and enjoy.

Nutrition:

Calories 165

Fat 11.2 g

Carbohydrates 5.2 g

Sugar 3.7 g

Protein 11.7 g

Cholesterol 327 mg

Crispy Breakfast Potatoes

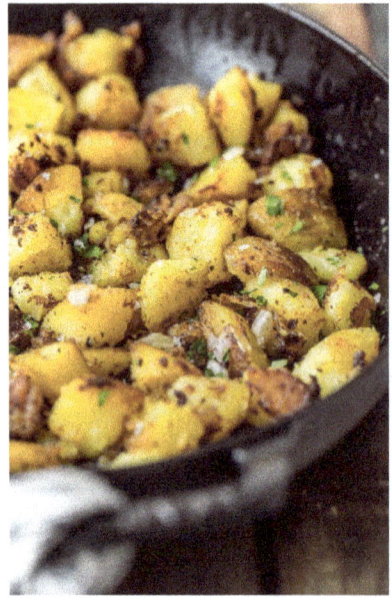

Preparation Time: 10 minutes

Cooking Time: 20 minutes

Servings: 6

Ingredients:

1 ½ lbs. potatoes, diced into ½-inch cubes

1 tsp paprika

1 tsp garlic powder

1 tbsp olive oil

½ tbsp dried parsley

¼ tsp chili powder

¼ tsp pepper

2 tsp salt

Directions:

Add potatoes into the mixing bowl. Add remaining ingredients over the potatoes and toss until evenly coated.

Arrange potatoes on air fryer oven tray and air fry at 400 F for 20 minutes. Turn potatoes to the other side halfway through.

Serve and enjoy.

Nutrition:

Calories 102

Fat 2.5 g

Carbohydrates 18.5 g

Sugar 1.5 g

Protein 2.1 g

Cholesterol 0 mg

Quick Cheese Omelet

Preparation Time: 5 minutes

Cooking Time: 9 minutes

Servings: 1

Ingredients:
2 eggs, lightly beaten
¼ cup cheddar cheese, shredded
¼ cup milk
Pepper
Salt
Directions:
In a bowl, whisk eggs with milk, pepper, and salt.

Spray small air fryer pan with cooking spray.

Pour egg mixture into the prepared pan and cook at 350 F for 6 minutes.

Sprinkle cheese on top and cook for 3 minutes more.

Serve and enjoy.

Nutrition:

Calories 270

Fat 19.4 g

Carbohydrates 4.1 g

Sugar 3.6 g

Protein 20.1 g

Cholesterol 362 mg

Tomato Spinach Frittata

Preparation Time: 10 minutes

Cooking Time: 7 minutes

Servings: 1

Ingredients:

2 eggs, lightly beaten

¼ cup spinach, chopped

¼ cup tomatoes, chopped

2 tbsp milk

1 tbsp parmesan cheese, grated

Pepper

Salt

Directions:

In a medium bowl, whisk eggs. Add remaining ingredients and whisk until well combined.

Spray small air fryer pan with cooking spray.

Pour egg mixture into the prepared pan and cook at 330 F for 7 minutes.

Serve and enjoy.

Nutrition:

Calories 189

Fat 11.7 g

Carbohydrates 4.3 g

Sugar 3.3 g

Protein 15.7 g

Cholesterol 337 mg

Roasted Brussels Sprouts & Sweet Potatoes

Preparation Time: 10 minutes

Cooking Time: 20 minutes

Servings: 4

Ingredients:

1 lb. Brussels sprouts, cut in half

2 sweet potatoes, wash and cut into 1-inch pieces

2 tbsp olive oil

¼ tsp garlic powder

½ tsp pepper

1 tsp salt

Directions:

Add sweet potatoes and Brussels sprouts in the mixing bowl.

Add remaining ingredients over sweet potatoes and Brussels sprouts and toss until well coated.

Transfer sweet potatoes and Brussels sprouts on air fryer oven tray and roast at 400 F for 10 minutes.

Turn sweet potatoes and Brussels sprouts to the other side and roast for 10 minutes more.

Serve and enjoy.

Nutrition:
Calories 138
Fat 7.4 g
Carbohydrates 17.2 g
Sugar 3.9 g
Protein 4.4 g
Cholesterol 0 mg

Roasted Potato wedges

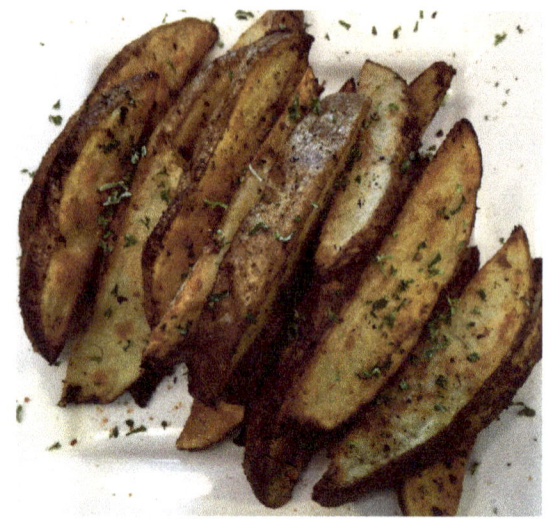

Preparation Time: 10 minutes

Cooking Time: 10 minutes

Servings: 6

Ingredients:

2 lbs. potatoes, cut into wedges

2 tbsp McCormick's chipotle seasoning

¼ cup olive oil

Directions:

Add potato wedges into the mixing bowl.

Add remaining ingredients over potato wedges and toss until well coated.

Transfer potato wedges onto the air fryer oven tray roast at 400 F for 5 minutes.

Turn potato wedges to the other side and roast for 5 minutes more.

Serve and enjoy.

Nutrition:
Calories 176
Fat 8.6 g
Carbohydrates 23.8 g
Sugar 1.7 g
Protein 2.5 g
Cholesterol 0 mg

Breakfast Egg Bites

Preparation Time: 10 minutes

Cooking Time: 13 minutes

Servings: 4

Ingredients:

4 eggs, lightly beaten

¼ cup ham, diced

¼ cup cheddar cheese, shredded

¼ cup bell pepper, diced

½ cup milk

Pepper

Salt

Directions:

Add all ingredients into the mixing bowl and whisk until well combined.

Spray muffin silicone mold with cooking spray.

Pour egg mixture into the silicone muffin mold and place it in the air fryer oven and bake at 350 F for 10 minutes.

After 10 minutes flip egg bites and cook for 3 minutes more.

Serve and enjoy.

Nutrition:
Calories 123
Fat 8.1 g
Carbohydrates 2.8 g
Sugar 2.1 g
Protein 9.8 g
Cholesterol 178 mg

Mains

Pumpkin and Pork Escallops

Preparation Time: 10 minutes

Cooking Time: 40 minutes

Servings: 4

Ingredients:

40 oz pork, ground

1 medium-sized pumpkin, cut into eighths

4 tbsp. dried sage

2 tbsp. clarified and unsalted butter

2 teaspoons dried thyme

2 teaspoons ground cinnamon

1 cup of fish broth

1 teaspoon of salt

1 teaspoon pepper

Directions:

Fix your Instant Pot to sauté mode and melt the unsalted butter or use the skillet to melt the butter and then pour in your Instant Pot.

Put all the spices in a bowl. Flavor the pork with the spices mix. Form the pork escallops. Add them into the Instant Pot.

Then, add in the pumpkin and pour in the fish broth.

Make sure to lock the lid and set on a HIGH pressure for 40 minutes.

Quick-release the pressure and transfer the pork escallops to a plate.

Combine the pumpkin with the pork escallops and ladle up the sauce (if any) all over the meat.

Nutrition:

Calories – 254

Protein – 57 g.

Fat – 63 g.

Carbs – 199 g.

Pork Curry with Cheese

Preparation Time: 15 minutes

Cooking Time: 40 minutes

Servings: 4

Ingredients:

20 oz pork, cubed

1 cup of champignons, sliced up

1 cup of Parmesan cheese, grated

1 medium onion, peeled and chopped

2 garlic cloves, minced

1 green chili, seeded and diced

1 tablespoon ginger

½ a tablespoon turmeric

1 cup of vegetable stock

3 tablespoons red curry paste

2 teaspoons salt

1 teaspoon cumin

½ teaspoon curry powder

¼ teaspoon ground fenugreek

¼ teaspoon black pepper

1 tablespoon tomato paste

3 tablespoons freshly squeezed lemon juice

1 cup of spinach, chopped

Directions:

Set the pot to sauté mode and add the champignons to the inner pot to cook for 10 minutes.

Add in the onion and mix well, cook until clear and caramelized.

Add the chili, garlic, ginger, turmeric and sauté for 1-2 minutes.

Add all the remaining ingredients and cancel the sauté mode.

Be sure to cover the lid and cook on a HIGH pressure for around 40 minutes.

Naturally release the pressure.

Stir in the tomato paste, spinach and lemon juice.

Portion the curry into four bowls or mugs and dollop each bowl with the grated Parmesan cheese.

Nutrition:

Calories – 247

Protein – 35 g.

Fat – 45 g.

Carbs – 213 g.

Lemon and Pork Chops in Tomato Sauce

Preparation Time: 15 minutes
Cooking Time: 45 minutes
Servings: 3
Ingredients:

5 pieces 2-inch pork

1 cup of tomato sauce

1 lemon, diced

4 ounces pancetta, diced

2 teaspoons pepper

2 carrots, peeled and chopped

1 orange peeled and diced

1 medium shallot, chopped

1 tablespoon lemon zest, minced

3 teaspoons dried rosemary

4 teaspoons garlic, minced

½ cup of lemon juice

¼ cup of chicken broth

soy sauce, to taste

Directions:

In a bowl, combine the pepper, lemon zest, dried rosemary and garlic. Toss the pork in the spices mix and pour the lemon juice over the meat. Then set the pork aside to marinate it for a couple of hours at room temperature or place in the fridge overnight.

Put all ingredients in your Instant Pot and close the lid to let them cook on a HIGH pressure for about 45 minutes. Release the pressure quickly and transfer the chops to a carving board.

Slice up the meat into strips. Divide into three plates and pour the soy sauce on top to serve.

Nutrition:

Calories – 382

Protein – 74 g.

Fat – 80 g.

Carbs – 284 g.

Buckwheat with Pork Chunks

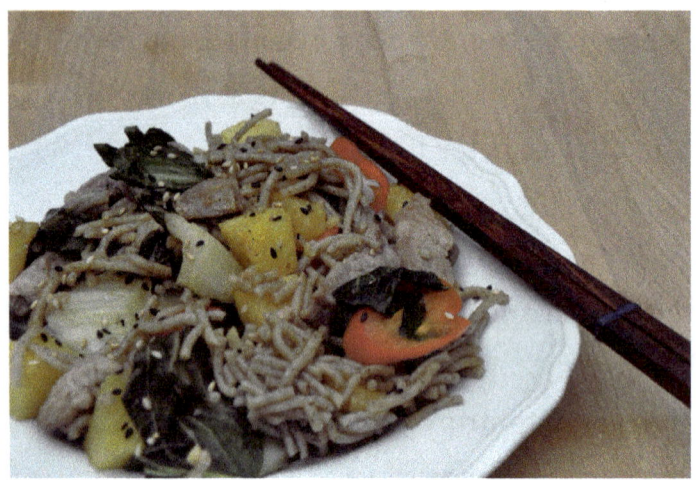

Preparation Time: 10 minutes

Cooking Time: 30 minutes

Servings: 4

Ingredients:

28 oz (1 can) pork chunks with broth, canned

1 cup of buckwheat, rinsed

4 medium onions, peeled and sliced

3 cups of water

½ teaspoon salt and pepper

Directions:

Immerse the buckwheat in the warm water for around 10 minutes. Then add in the buckwheat to your pot.

In a skillet or wok, fry the onions for 10 minutes until clear and caramelized. In a bowl, mash the pork using a fork.

Combine the buckwheat, pork chunks and caramelized onions and add to your Instant Pot.

Make sure to lock the lid and cook on a HIGH pressure for 20 minutes.

Naturally release the pressure over 10 minutes.

Portion the buckwheat and pork chunks into four deep containers and dollop each bowl with the salt and pepper.

Serve the buckwheat porridge and pork chunks with the coffee.

Nutrition:

Calories – 285

Protein – 52 g.

Fat – 79 g.

Carbs – 237 g.

Lime Pork with Pineapple and Peanuts

Preparation Time: 10 minutes
Cooking Time: 45 minutes
Servings: 4
Ingredients:

20 oz pork

1 cup of pineapple, diced

1 cup of peanuts

2 tablespoons soy sauce

1 tablespoon dry basil

5 garlic cloves, minced

4 tablespoons olive oil

Salt as needed

4 tablespoons freshly squeezed lime juice

½ tablespoon of corn starch

½ cup of water

Directions:

Marinate the pork in the salt, soy sauce, dry basil, minced garlic and lime juice for at least few hours at room temperature or place in the fridge overnight.

Preheat the oven to 240°-260°F and roast the peanuts in the oven for 10 minutes until crispy and then let it cool completely. Then grind the peanuts using a food processor or blender.

Add the marinated pork and all the listed ingredients to your Instant Pot.

Make sure to lock the lid and set the timer to 45 minutes and cook the pork on a MEAT/STEW mode.

Naturally release the pressure over 10 minutes.

Portion the pork into four deep containers and dollop each bowl with the salt and pepper. Serve the pork with the tea.

Nutrition:

Calories – 374

Protein – 62 g.

Fat – 72 g.

Carbs – 271 g.

Pork in Tomato Sauce with Pineapple

Preparation Time: 15 minutes

Cooking Time: 55 minutes

Servings: 3

Ingredients:

5 pieces 2-inch pork

1 cup of pineapple, cubed

1 cup of tomato sauce

4 ounces pancetta, diced

2 teaspoons pepper

2 carrots, peeled and chopped

3 teaspoons dried rosemary

4 teaspoons garlic, minced

½ cup of orange juice

¼ cup of chicken broth

soy sauce, to taste

Directions:

Combine the pepper, dried rosemary and garlic in a bowl. Toss the pork in the spices mix. Then set the pork aside to marinate it for at least few hours or place in the fridge overnight.

Put all ingredients to your Instant Pot and secure the lid to let itcook for about 55 minutes on a HIGH pressure.

Release the pressure quickly and transfer the pork to a carving board.

Slice up the meat into strips. Divide into three plates and pour the soy sauce on top to serve.

Nutrition:

Calories – 382

Protein – 74 g.

Fat – 82 g.

Carbs – 286 g.

Pork in Tomato Sauce with Butter

Preparation Time: 15 minutes

Cooking Time: 45 minutes

Servings: 4

Ingredients:

5 pieces 2-inch pork

1 cup of tomato sauce

4 tablespoons salted butter

5 garlic cloves, minced

3 teaspoons dried rosemary

2 teaspoons black pepper

1 teaspoon nutmeg

1 cup of chicken broth

Directions:

In a bowl, mix the dried rosemary, nutmeg, black pepper, and garlic. Toss the pork in the spices mix. Then set the pork aside to marinate it for a couple of hours at room temperature or place in the fridge overnight.

Put all the ingredients in your Instant Pot and close the lid to let them cook on a HIGH pressure for about 45 minutes.

Release the pressure and place the pork to a carving board.

Slice up the meat into strips and then divide into four bowls or plates and ladle up the tomato sauce and then spoon some salted butter on top to serve with the white bread and wine.

Nutrition:

Calories – 393

Protein – 89 g.

Fat – 92 g.

Carbs – 293 g.

Pork with Lemon

Preparation Time: 10 minutes

Cooking Time: 45 minutes

Servings: 3

Ingredients:

20 oz pork

2 lemons, peeled and diced

5 tablespoons liquid honey

2 tablespoon Gouda cheese, grated

2 tablespoons soy sauce

1 tablespoon dry basil

5 garlic cloves, minced

4 tablespoons olive oil

Salt as needed

1 cup of freshly squeezed lemon juice

½ tablespoon of corn starch

½ cup of water

Directions:

Marinate the pork in the salt, soy sauce, dry basil, minced garlic, lemon juice and honey for a couple of hours at room temperature or place in the fridge overnight. Add the marinated pork and all other ingredients to your Instant Pot.

Secure the lid, fix the timer to 45 minutes and cook the pork on MEAT/STEW option.

Naturally release the pressure for 10 minutes.

Serve and enjoy!

Nutrition:

Calories – 379

Protein – 64 g.

Fat – 74 g.

Carbs – 277 g.

Spicy Pork Shoulder with Brown Rice

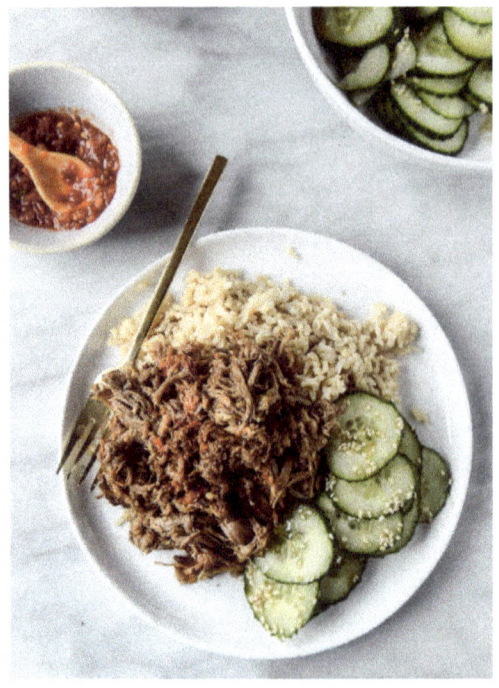

Preparation Time: 10 minute

Cooking Time: 65 minutes

Servings: 4

Ingredients:

1 cup of brown rice

30 oz pork shoulder, cut into half

1 tablespoon liquid smoke

5 tablespoons sunflower oil

1 cup of water

2 teaspoons chili pepper powder

salt and pepper to taste

brown rice or steamed green beans for serving (optional)

Directions:

Wash the brown rice several times and let the water boil to cook the rice for about 20 minutes. Add 2 tablespoons sunflower oil when the rice is ready.

Fix your Instant Pot to sauté mode and pour some oil to heat it up.

Add in the pork, salt, chili pepper powder and pepper, brown each side for 5 minutes until the both sides are slightly browned. Transfer them to a plate.

Put the water and liquid smoke to the Instant Pot and place the meat and spoon the rice.

Make sure to lock the lid and cook for60 minutes on a HIGH pressure, release pressure naturally over 10 minutes.

Transfer the pork meat to the cutting board and shred using 2 forks. Portion the pork into four plates and dollop each plate with the cooking liquid. Serve it with the rice or green beans on the side.

Nutrition:

Calories – 384,Protein – 64 g. Fat – 75 g., Carbs – 275 g.

Conclusion

When you are on a diet trying to lose weight or manage a condition, you will be strictly confined to follow an eating plan. Such plans often place numerous demands on individuals: food may need to be boiled, other foods are forbidden, permitting you only to eat small portions and so on.

On the other hand, a lifestyle such as the Mediterranean diet is entirely stress-free. It is easy to follow because there are almost no restrictions. There is no time limit on the Mediterranean diet because it is more of a lifestyle than a diet. You do not need to stop at some point but carry on for the rest of your life. The foods that you eat under the Mediterranean model include unrefined cereals, white meats, and the occasional dairy products.

The Mediterranean lifestyle, unlike other diets, also requires you to engage with family and friends and share meals together. It has been noted that communities around the Mediterranean spend between one and two hours enjoying their meals. This kind of bonding between family members or friends helps bring people closer together, which helps foster closer bonds hence fewer cases of depression, loneliness, or stress, all of which are precursors to chronic diseases.

You will achieve many benefits using the Instant Pot Pressure Cooker. These are just a few instances you will discover in your Mediterranean-style recipes:

Pressure cooking means that you can (on average) cook meals 75% faster than boiling/braising on the stovetop or baking and roasting in a conventional oven.

This is especially helpful for vegan meals that entail the use of dried beans, legumes, and pulses. Instead of pre-soaking these ingredients for hours before use, you can pour them directly into the Instant Pot, add water, and pressure cook these for several minutes. However, always follow your recipe carefully since they have been tested for accuracy.

Nutrients are preserved. You can use your pressure-cooking techniques using the Instant Pot to ensure the heat is evenly and quickly distributed. It is not essential to immerse the food into the water. You will provide plenty of water in the cooker for efficient steaming. You will also be saving the essential vitamins and minerals. The food won't become oxidized by the exposure of air or heat. Enjoy those fresh green veggies with their natural and vibrant colors.

The cooking elements help keep the foods fully sealed, so the steam and aromas don't linger throughout your entire home. That is a plus, especially for items such as cabbage, which throws out a distinctive smell.

You will find that beans and whole grains will have a softer texture and will have an improved taste. The meal will be cooked consistently since the Instant Pot provides even heat distribution.

You'll also save tons of time and money. You will be using much less water, and the pot is fully insulated, making it more energy-efficient when compared to boiling or steaming your foods on the stovetop. It is also less expensive than using a microwave, not to mention how much more flavorful the food will be when prepared in the Instant Pot cooker.

You can delay the cooking of your food items so you can plan ahead of time. You won't need to stand around as you await your meal. You can reduce the cooking time by reducing the 'hands-on' time. Just leave for work or a day of activities, and you will come home to a special treat. In a nutshell, the Instant Pot is:

Easy To Use

Healthy recipes for the entire family are provided.

You can make authentic one-pot recipes in your Instant Pot.

If you forget to switch on your slow cooker, you can make any meal done in a few minutes in your Instant Pot.

You can securely and smoothly cook meat from frozen.

It's a laid-back way to cook. You don't have to watch a pan on the stove or a pot in the oven.

The pressure cooking procedure develops delicious flavors swiftly.

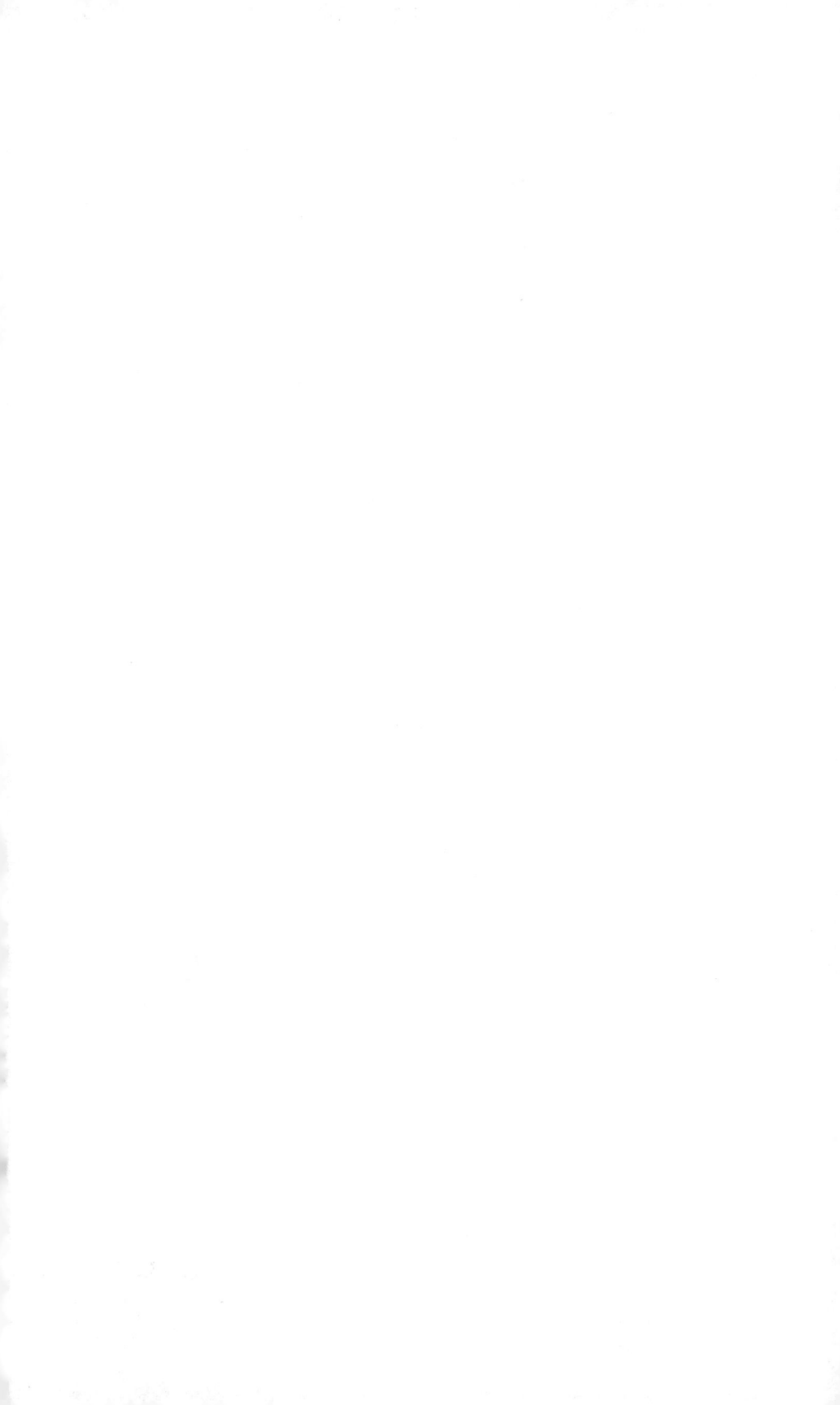

CPSIA information can be obtained
at www.ICGtesting.com
Printed in the USA
BVHW051011060421
604323BV00002B/45